ST/ESA/SER.A/157

Department for Economic and Social Information and Policy Analysis
Population Division

Reproductive Rights and Reproductive Health: A Concise Report

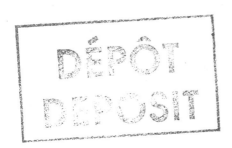

 United Nations   New York, 1996

NOTE

The designations employed and the presentation of the material in the present report do not imply the expression of any opinion whatsoever on the part of the Secretariat of the United Nations concerning the legal status of any country, territory, city or area or of its authorities, or concerning the delimitation of its frontiers or boundaries.

The term "country" as used in the text and tables of this report also refers, as appropriate, to territories or areas.

The designations "developed" and "developing" economies are intended for statistical convenience and do not necessarily express a judgement about the stage reached by a particular country or area in the development process.

The report has been edited in accordance with United Nations practice and requirements.

ST/ESA/SER.A/157

UN 2
ST/ESA/SER.A/157

UNITED NATIONS PUBLICATION

Sales No. E.96.XIII. 11

ISBN 92-1-151307-3

PREFACE

The present report has been prepared in response to Economic and Social Council resolution 1995/55, in which the Council endorsed the terms of reference and the topic-oriented and prioritized multi-year work programme proposed by the Commission on Population and Development in its report on its twenty-eighth session. According to the multi-year work programme, which would serve as a framework for the assessment of the progress achieved in the implementation of the Programme of Action of the International Conference on Population and Development, a new series of reports on a special set of themes would be prepared annually. The theme selected for 1996, "Reproductive rights and reproductive health, including population information, education and communication", is the topic of the present report. The following are the topics for succeeding years:

1997: International migration, with special emphasis on the linkages between migration and development, and on gender issues and the family;

1998: Health and mortality, with special emphasis on the linkages between health and development, and on gender and age;

1999: Population growth, structure and distribution, with special emphasis on sustained economic growth and sustainable development, including education.

The present report provides a summary of recent information on selected aspects of reproductive rights and reproductive health and covers such topics as entry into reproductive life; reproductive behaviour; contraception; abortion; maternal mortality and morbidity; sexually transmitted diseases, including HIV/AIDS; reproductive rights; and population information, education and communication with respect to reproductive rights and reproductive health.

The current report was prepared by the Population Division of the Department for Economic and Social Information and Policy Analysis of the United Nations Secretariat. Acknowledgements are due to the various United Nations offices, regional commissions and specialized agencies that helped directly or indirectly in the preparation of the report: chapters V and VI were prepared by the World Health Organization (WHO); and chapter VIII was based on contributions from the United Nations Children's Fund (UNICEF), the United Nations Population Fund (UNFPA), the United Nations Educational, Scientific and Cultural Organization (UNESCO) and WHO.

CONTENTS

TABLES

FIGURES

Explanatory notes

Symbols of United Nations documents are composed of capital letters combined with figures.

The following symbols have been used in the tables throughout this report:

Two dots (..) indicate that data are not available or are not separately reported.

An em dash (—) indicates that the amount is nil or negligible.

A hyphen (-) indicates that the item is not applicable.

A minus sign (–) before a figure indicates a decrease.

A point (.) is used to indicate decimals.

A slash (/) indicates a crop year or financial year, e.g., 1994/95.

Use of a hyphen (-) between dates representing years, e.g., 1994-1995, signifies the full period involved, including the beginning and end years.

Details and percentages in tables do not necessarily add to totals because of rounding.

Reference to "dollars" ($) indicates United States dollars, unless otherwise stated.

The term "billion" signifies a thousand million.

The group of least developed countries currently comprises 48 countries: Afghanistan, Angola, Bangladesh, Benin, Bhutan, Burkina Faso, Burundi, Cambodia, Cape Verde, Central African Republic, Chad, Comoros, Djibouti, Equatorial Guinea, Eritrea, Ethiopia, Gambia, Guinea, Guinea-Bissau, Haiti, Kiribati, Lao People's Democratic Republic, Lesotho, Liberia, Madagascar, Malawi, Maldives, Mali, Mauritania, Mozambique, Myanmar, Nepal, Niger, Rwanda, Samoa, Sao Tome and Principe, Sierra Leone, Solomon Islands, Somalia, Sudan, Togo, Tuvalu, Uganda, United Republic of Tanzania, Vanuatu, Yemen, Zaire and Zambia.

The following abbreviations have been used:

AIDS	acquired immunodeficiency syndrome
DHS	Demographic and Health Surveys
HIV	human immunodeficiency virus
IUD	intra-uterine device
RAMOS	Reproductive Age Mortality Surveys
UNESCO	United Nations Educational, Scientific and Cultural Organization
UNFPA	United Nations Population Fund
UNICEF	United Nations Children's Fund
WFS	World Fertility Survey
WHO	World Health Organization

INTRODUCTION

The Programme of Action of the International Conference on Population and Development, held at Cairo in September 1994, defines reproductive rights and reproductive health as follows:

"Reproductive health is a state of complete physical, mental and social well-being and not merely the absence of disease or infirmity, in all matters relating to the reproductive system and to its functions and processes. Reproductive health therefore implies that people are able to have a satisfying and safe sex life and that they have the capability to reproduce and the freedom to decide if, when and how often to do so. Implicit in this last condition are the right of men and women to be informed and to have access to safe, effective, affordable and acceptable methods of family planning of their choice, as well as other methods of their choice for regulation of fertility which are not against the law, and the right of access to appropriate health-care services that will enable women to go safely through pregnancy and childbirth and provide couples with the best chance of having a healthy infant. In line with the above definition of reproductive health, reproductive health care is defined as the constellation of methods, techniques and services that contribute to reproductive health and well-being by preventing and solving reproductive health problems. It also includes sexual health, the purpose of which is the enhancement of life and personal relations, and not merely counselling and care related to reproduction and sexually transmitted diseases.

"Bearing in mind the above definition, reproductive rights embrace certain human rights that are already recognized in national laws, international human rights documents and other consensus documents. These rights rest on the recognition of the basic right of all couples and individuals to decide freely and responsibly the number, spacing and timing of their children and to have the information and means to do so, and the right to attain the highest standard of sexual and reproductive health. It also includes their right to make decisions concerning reproduction free of discrimination, coercion and violence, as expressed in human rights documents. In the exercise of this right, they should take into account the needs of their living and future children and their responsibilities towards the community. The promotion of the responsible exercise of these rights for all people should be the fundamental basis for government- and community-supported policies and programmes in the area of reproductive health, including family planning. As part of their commitment, full attention should be given to the promotion of mutually respectful and equitable gender relations and particularly to meeting the educational and service needs of adolescents to enable them to deal in a positive and responsible way with their sexuality. Reproductive health eludes many of the world's people because of such factors as: inadequate levels of knowledge about human sexuality and inappropriate or poor-quality reproductive health information and services; the prevalence of high-risk sexual behaviour; discriminatory social practices; negative attitudes towards women and girls; and the limited power many women and girls have over their sexual and reproductive lives. Adolescents are particularly vulnerable because of their lack of information and access to relevant services in most countries. Older women and men have distinct reproductive and sexual health issues which are often inadequately addressed." (United Nations, 1995a, chap. VII, paras. 7.2-7.3)

The broad and comprehensive approach to reproductive health reflected in the above definitions contrasts with various previous approaches dealing with reproduction. The earlier approaches focused on specific aspects of reproductive health. For example, family planning programmes concentrated on providing information and services on contraception. Maternal and child health programmes focused on promoting the health of mothers and their young children, while safe motherhood programmes have emphasized the need to ensure that pregnant women receive adequate prenatal care, safe delivery and postnatal care and sought to address the high risks that women in many contexts face in relation to child-bearing.

Reproductive health incorporates all of those aspects in a comprehensive manner. While acknowledging the importance of family planning, the approach recognizes that reproductive health is not limited to the child-bearing ages and that reproductive health concerns men as well as women. It also recognizes that to address reproductive health issues successfully, there is need to address relevant social behaviour and cultural practices.

It is based on the premise that the health status of individuals at any given time is affected by their earlier experiences. The reproductive health of men and women of child-bearing age, for example, reflects not only their current experiences but also their health status during infancy, childhood and adolescence. Similarly, their health status beyond the reproductive ages may reflect their earlier reproductive experiences. The experiences of one generation also have implications for the health of the next generation.

The present report provides a global review of selected aspects of reproductive rights and reproductive health. The topics covered include entry into reproductive life; reproductive behaviour; contraception; abortion; maternal mortality and morbidity; sexually transmitted diseases, including human immunodeficiency virus (HIV) and the acquired immunodeficiency syndrome (AIDS); policy issues related to reproductive rights; and population information, education and communication with respect to reproductive rights and reproductive health.

To the extent possible, the reproductive rights and reproductive health of both men and women are reviewed. However, data collection and research have until recently focused primarily on the reproductive and contraceptive behaviour of women. It is only during the past few years that demographic and health surveys have begun to include samples of men. The need to collect data and conduct research on the reproductive attitudes and behaviour of both men and women has become more imperative, given the renewed emphasis on the shared responsibility of partners in matters related to reproduction. Information is also lacking on the reproductive health of adolescents and of older men and women, which are usually not the subject of inquiry in demographic and health surveys.

I. ENTRY INTO REPRODUCTIVE LIFE

Initiation of reproductive capability generally occurs in the second decade of life. The events which define entry into reproductive life, and their timing, are important determinants of both fertility and reproductive health and have important implications for the future life course of individuals. The stage of life during which individuals reach sexual maturity has come to be known as adolescence; it is the period of transition from childhood to adulthood. Although the change is biological, the duration and nature of adolescence is primarily a social construct and thus varies greatly from culture to culture. This review refers to the age range of 10-24 years but focuses mostly on age group 15-24, which the World Health Organization (WHO) refers to as "young people". Within this age span are found many of the variations noted between countries and population subgroups in the events that define the beginning of reproductive life.

Adolescence is a period of development that is increasingly recognized both as an important determinant of future health and as an especially vulnerable period of life. In particular, increasing concern is being expressed about sexual risk-taking among young people and the consequences of such behaviour as teenage pregnancy and the incidence of sexually transmitted diseases, including HIV. The challenges of addressing the needs of adolescents are compounded by demographic factors. It has been estimated that in 1995 young people made up over 14 per cent of the total population in the more developed regions and almost 20 per cent in the less developed regions (see table 1).

In a number of societies, menarche signifies maturity and the readiness to marry or commence sexual activity. Studies documenting the age at menarche show that the age of onset varies by approximately five years between different population groups. The average age for each region indicates a younger age at onset in the more developed than in the less developed regions. Age at menarche has fallen in most developed countries. In developing countries, the decline is less well documented, but there is some evidence of a fall in age at onset in a number of population groups. The fall in age at menarche implies an earlier potential to reproduce. However, in general, it would appear that the effect of this biological factor has been offset by other influences, especially by increases in age at first marriage.

Traditionally, age at marriage has been regarded as marking the initiation of sexual activity and, therefore, the beginning of exposure to reproduction. Changes in the timing of first marriage around the world

4

TABLE 1. ESTIMATED AND PROJECTED POPULATION AGED 15-24 YEARS,
1995 AND 2025

		1995		2025	
Region	Sex	Population aged 15-24	Percentage of total population	Population aged 15-24	Percentage of total population
World	Total	1 028 054	18.0	1 306 410	15.8
	Male	526 795	18.2	666 888	16.0
	Female	501 259	17.6	639 522	15.5
More developed regions	Male	83 838	14.8	73 634	12.2
	Female	80 245	13.4	70 161	11.1
Less developed regions[b]	Male	442 957	19.1	593 254	16.6
	Female	421 013	18.8	569 360	16.3
Africa	Male	70 315	19.4	147 028	19.7
	Female	69 599	19.1	145 226	19.4
Asia	Male	334 080	18.9	395 455	15.7
	Female	313 141	18.5	374 689	15.3
Europe	Male	52 357	14.9	41 442	11.9
	Female	50 167	13.3	39 409	10.7
Latin America and the Caribbean	Male	47 353	19.7	56 220	15.9
	Female	46 656	19.2	54 639	15.3
Northern America . . .	Male	20 310	14.2	23 762	13.1
	Female	19 433	13.0	22 728	12.1
Oceania	Male	2 377	16.5	2 979	14.5
	Female	2 262	15.9	2 829	13.8

Source: World Population Prospects: The 1994 Revision (United Nations publication, Sales No. E.95.XIII.6).

[a]More developed regions comprise all regions in Europe, Northern America and Australia, New Zealand and Japan.

[b]Less developed regions comprise all regions of Africa, Asia (excluding Japan), Latin America and the Caribbean, and regions of Melanesia, Micronesia and Polynesia.

are well documented, and it is clear that age at first marriage among women has risen dramatically in many countries. In the developing countries with data from the Demographic and Health Surveys (DHS), changes in the age at marriage can be examined by comparing the experience of women in different cohorts (see table 2). The surveys use a broad definition of marriage which includes both formalized and informal unions.[1] The data indicate that the proportion married by age 20 among young women (those aged 20-24 at the time of the survey) is considerably lower than that among older women (aged 40-44 at the

5

time of the survey) in nearly all the developing countries surveyed. The shift towards later marriage is most pronounced in the Asian countries: taking the average for eight countries shows that 57 per cent of women currently aged 40-44 years first married before age 20; the corresponding figure for women currently aged 20-24 years is 37 per cent. In Africa, the reduction in the average proportion married by age 20 has been almost as sharp—from 72 to 55 per cent—but the prevalence of teenage marriage remains much higher than in Asia. In Latin America and the Caribbean, changes in the timing of first marriage have been more modest, and the average proportion married before age 20 (42 per cent) is somewhat higher than in Asia.

Age at marriage for women has also risen in the past 20 years in the developed countries, although the information on trends is not comparable with that for developing countries because most data derived from civil registration deal with legal marriage only (see table 3). In 1970, the typical average age at first marriage in Northern and Western Europe was 22-24 years. By 1990, age at marriage in many countries in Northern and Western Europe had risen to 25-27 years. Increases are also observed in Japan and in Northern America. In Eastern and Southern Europe changes in marriage ages have been more modest.

In most countries there is a general trend towards later marriage with increased educational level. Urban or rural residence represents a further influence on marriage ages for women. DHS data show that women with at least 10 years of education marry between two and seven years later than those with less than primary education. Women living in urban areas typically marry later than their rural counterparts, although the urban/rural gap varies considerably. In many developing countries, there is a 20 per cent or larger difference in the proportion marrying by age 20. In others, the difference is small.

Differences in the age at marriage between men and women have narrowed over time in many countries in Africa, most notably in Northern Africa, Asia and many countries in Latin America and the Caribbean. The convergence has been most marked in countries where differences were the largest. In Northern America and Europe, the gaps between the sexes have contracted further in recent decades.

In many European countries, the upward trend in age at marriage has coincided with an increase in the proportion cohabiting. The age-specific proportions of women who are living in consensual unions for seven European countries in 1985-1990 are shown in figure I. At ages 15-19, the proportions cohabiting range from nearly 0 to 20 per cent. The prevalence of cohabitation peaks at ages 20-24, with a range of approximately 10-40 per cent, and declines thereafter. The major reason for the decline in informal cohabitation after age 25 is the growing

TABLE 2. MEDIAN AGE AT FIRST MARRIAGE AND PERCENTAGE OF WOMEN MARRIED BEFORE THE AGE OF 20 AMONG RESPONDENTS AGED 20-24 AND 40-44 YEARS AT THE TIME OF THE SURVEY, SELECTED DEVELOPING COUNTRIES

Region and country	Year of survey	Median age at first marriage		Percentage married before 20	
		20-24	40-44	20-24	40-44
Africa					
Botswana	1988	..	23.5	19	33
Burundi	1987	20.5	19.4	44	58
Cameroon	1991	..	..	73	85
Egypt	1988-1989	20.8	17.8	46	67
Ghana	1988	18.7	17.6	63	77
Kenya	1989	19.8	17.4	52	75
Liberia	1986	18.2	16.0	64	81
Mali	1987	15.9	15.6	92	90
Morocco	1987	..	16.8	36	78
Namibia	1992	..	..	20	28
Niger	1992	..	..	90	94
Nigeria	1990	17.8	16.8	68	71
Senegal	1986	..	..	70	86
Sudan	1989-1990	..	15.8	37	78
Togo	1988	18.6	18.0	63	69
Tunisia	1988	..	19.4	21	54
Uganda	1988-1989	17.8	16.6	73	83
United Rep. of Tanzania	1991-1992	..	..	61	76
Zambia	1992	..	..	64	81
Zimbabwe	1988-1989	19.7	18.1	53	69
Asia					
China	1987-1988	..	..	20	48
Indonesia	1987	19.8	16.4	51	80
Jordan	1990	..	18.9	30	62
Pakistan	1990-1991	..	18.5	49	61
Philippines	1993	..	..	29	38
Sri Lanka	1987	..	21.4	28	41
Thailand	1986	22.9	20.2	37	48
Turkey	1988	..	..	50	75
Latin America and the Caribbean					
Belize	1981	21.0	20.1	44	50
Bolivia	1989	21.4	20.7	41	43
Brazil	1986	21.5	20.7	40	44
Colombia	1990	21.8[a]	20.9	37	42

7

TABLE 2 (*continued*)

Region and country	Year of survey	Median age at first marriage		Percentage married before 20	
		20-24	40-44	20-24	40-44
Latin America and the Caribbean (*continued*)					
Costa Rica	1986	18.7	21.0	40	39
Dominican Republic	1991	19.2	18.4	47	63
Ecuador	1987	20.7	19.9	44	51
El Salvador	1985	..	19.3	59	58
Guatemala	1987	18.9	19.1	60	56
Haiti	1989	..	..	15	..
Jamaica	1989	16.2	17.9	39	65
Mexico	1987	20.9	19.7	44	53
Paraguay	1990	..	20.6	41	44
Peru	1991-1992	23.3[a]	20.6	31	45
Trinidad and Tobago	1987	19.7	19.8	53	52

Source: Bryant Robey and others, *The Reproductive Revolution: New Survey Findings,* Population Reports, Series M, No. 11 (Baltimore, Maryland, The Johns Hopkins School of Hygiene and Public Health, Population Information Program, 1992).
[a]Estimate from Demographic and Health Surveys carried out in 1988

TABLE 3. MEAN AGE OF WOMEN AT FIRST MARRIAGE, SELECTED COUNTRIES OF EUROPE AND NORTHERN AMERICA, 1970-1992

Region and country	1970	1975	1980	1985	1990	1992
Asia						
Japan	24.2	27.4	25.2	25.5	25.9	26.0
Eastern Europe						
Bulgaria	21.7	21.8	21.7	21.9	21.7	21.9
Czech Republic . . .	21.6	21.6	21.5	21.6	21.5	..
Hungary	21.2	20.8	21.3	21.3	21.5	21.6
Poland	21.9	20.8	21.3	21.3	21.5	21.6
Romania	..	21.5	22.0	22.0	22.0	22.1
Russian Federation						
Slovak Republic . . .	22.2	22.5	22.7	22.8	22.0	21.2
Northern Europe						
Denmark	22.8	23.7	24.8	26.3	27.6	28.2
Estonia	24.8	24.0	23.2	23.2	23.0	..
Finland	23.0	23.5	24.5	25.4	26.5	26.9
Iceland	23.2	22.7	23.2	24.9	26.1	..

8

TABLE 3 *(continued)*

Region and country	1970	1975	1980	1985	1990	1992
Northern Europe *(continued)*						
Ireland	24.8	24.4	24.1	25.0	25.9	..
Latvia	..	..	..	22.7	22.2	22.4
Norway	22.7	22.9	23.6	24.4	26.2	..
Sweden	24.0	25.1	26.4	27.5	27.6	27.8
United Kingdom . . .	22.4	22.8	23.0	23.8	25.2	..
Southern Europe						
Bosnia-Herzegovina .	..	..	22.0	22.4	23.3	..
Croatia	21.8	22.1	22.4	22.6	23.2	..
Greece	22.9	22.8	22.3	22.8	23.8	24.4
Italy	24.1	24.0	24.1	24.5	25.6	..
Malta	..	..	24.7	22.5	..	..
Portugal	24.3	23.7	23.3	23.6	24.2	24.5
San Marino	22.6	22.1	24.1	24.8	24.9	25.1
Slovenia	23.6	22.2	22.3	21.3	23.6	24.1
Spain	24.7	23.4	23.4	24.2	25.3	..
The former Yugoslav Rep. of Macedonia	..	..	22.2	22.4	22.8	..
Yugoslavia (former)						
Montenegro	..	..	23.1	23.4	24.2	..
Serbia	..	..	23.0	23.2	23.7	..
Western Europe						
Austria	23.1	22.8	23.1	24.0	25.1	25.7
Belgium	22.4	21.6	22.3	23.1	24.6	24.9
France	22.4	22.5	23.0	24.3	24.7	26.1
Germany[a]	23.0	22.7	23.4	24.6	25.9	26.5
Germany[b]	21.9	21.3	21.3	22.2	23.7	25.1
Liechtenstein	23.1	25.1	25.6	26.0	..	..
Luxembourg	23.2	23.3	23.0	24.1	25.4	25.9
Netherlands	22.8	22.6	23.1	24.4	25.9	26.6
Switzerland	24.2	24.3	25.2	26.1	27.0	27.3
Northern America						
Canada	22.7	22.5	23.3	24.6	26.1	..
United States of America	20.6	20.8	21.8	23.0	..	..

Source: Japan, Ministry of Health and Welfare, *Latest Demographic Statistics, 1995* (Tokyo, 1995), table b-12; Council of Europe, *Recent Demographic Developments in Europe, 1994* (Strasbourg, France, 1994), table 2.3.

[a]Former Federal Republic of Germany.
[b]Former German Democratic Republic.

9

Percentage

Figure 1. Percentage of women living in consensual union, by age, selected European countries, 1985-1990

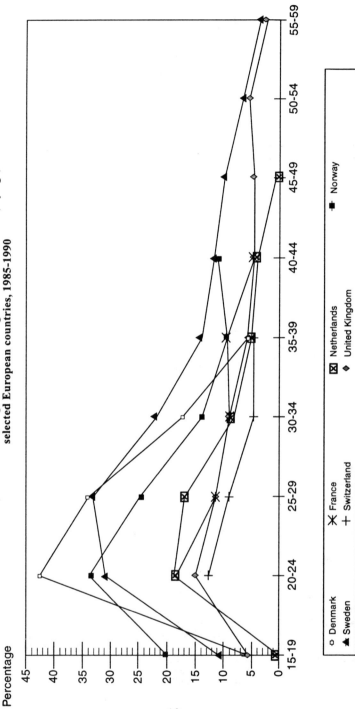

Legend:
- □ Denmark
- ✕ France
- ⊠ Netherlands
- ■ Norway
- ▲ Sweden
- + Switzerland
- ◆ United Kingdom

Source: European Commission, *The Demographic Situation in the European Union: 1994 Report* (Srrasbourg, France, 1994), graph 21.

dominance of legal marriage. In most European countries, marriage remains the norm at peak child-bearing ages.

Delays in the timing of first marriage have played a key role in the fertility decline in many countries because most births continue to occur within marriage. Increases in the age at marriage, however, do not necessarily translate into a shortening of the reproductive life span. Premarital births are increasing in a number of countries around the world. Furthermore, the prevalence of sexually transmitted diseases among unmarried adolescents suggests that premarital sexual activity is not uncommon and may be increasing.

A growing body of survey data reveals wide variability in sexual behaviour among young people. In some areas of the world sexual activity begins early and is frequently premarital, while in others it is dictated by strong social sanctions and commonly coincides with marriage, although this, too, may occur at a very early age. Despite the paucity of systematic data and the variability in sexual behaviour of young people, some broad patterns emerge from the evidence.

In most areas of the world, men report an earlier age at sexual initiation than women, a greater number of partners and a longer period of time between sexual initiation and marriage. They are more likely than women to report premarital sexual activity. Age differences between partners have important implications for the transmission of sexually transmitted diseases. Men typically have younger female partners, which increases the vulnerability of younger women to sexually transmitted diseases and HIV infection. Relations between older men and younger women are reported to be increasingly common in some parts of Africa.

In the industrialized countries, there are indications of an increase in the overall proportion of young people who are sexually active. Age at marriage has increased; there is evidence of a fall in the age at sexual initiation, and a greater proportion of adolescents are involved in cohabiting relations.

In sub-Saharan Africa and Latin America and the Caribbean, age at sexual initiation appears to have remained unchanged, although sexual activity begins at an early age in many countries. Increases in age at marriage, in the absence of changes in age at sexual initiation, have meant that more young people have been exposed to premarital sexual activity.

Little is known about the sexual behaviour of young people in Asia. It is typically assumed that premarital sexual activity is uncommon and subject to strong societal constraints. Evidence is sparse, but a few studies indicate that sexual initiation coincides with marriage for the majority of young women, or is a prelude to marriage. Thus, any rise in age at marriage will also increase the age at sexual initiation.

11

II. REPRODUCTIVE BEHAVIOUR

The current total fertility rate (TFR) for the world as a whole is estimated to be 3.1 children per woman (see table 4). This average, however, conceals a large diversity between and within regions. The gap between the more developed regions (TFR of 1.7) and the less developed regions (TFR of 3.5), although narrower than in the past, remains sizeable. The highest TFR is observed in Africa (5.8), followed by Latin America and the Caribbean (3.1) and Asia (3.0). At the country level, current fertility rates range from 7.6 in Yemen to 1.2 in Italy and Spain.

During the past decade, fertility has continued its downward trend. At the world level, the average number of children per woman declined from 3.6 in 1980-1985 to 3.1 in 1990-1995. The underlying change in reproductive behaviour, however, differs greatly by region. In the more developed regions, fertility, which has been below replacement since the late 1970s, experienced only a slight decline, whereas in the less developed regions fertility fell from 4.2 to 3.5. The observed reduction was more modest in the least developed countries, where fertility declined from 6.4 to 5.8 children.

In recent decades, adolescent child-bearing has emerged as an issue of increasing concern throughout the developing and the developed world. There is a growing awareness that early child-bearing poses a health risk for the mother and the child and may truncate a girl's educational career, threatening her economic prospects, earning capacity and overall well-being.

It is estimated that worldwide about 15 million girls aged 15-19 give birth each year and that about 11 per cent of all babies are currently born to adolescents (United Nations, 1995b). There is, however, considerable variation across regions. The level of adolescent fertility in the least developed countries (140 births per 1,000 women under age 20) is twice as high as that in developing countries (65 births per 1,000) and four times higher than that in the developed countries (32 births per 1,000). In the developing regions, adolescent fertility rates are highest in Africa (136 births per 1,000), followed by Latin America and the Caribbean (79 births per 1,000) and lowest in Asia (45 births per 1,000). In many societies, a pattern of early marriage contributes to elevated rates of child-bearing among adolescents. Although several countries have raised the legal age at marriage, this measure has had only limited impact in traditional societies where early marriage and child-bearing have long been promoted by social and cultural mores.

12

TABLE 4. TOTAL FERTILITY RATES, WORLD, MAJOR AREAS AND REGIONS, 1980-1985, 1985-1990 AND 1990-1995[a]

Major area and region	Total fertility rate[b]		
	1980-1985	1985-1990	1990-1995
World total	3.6	3.4	3.1
More developed regions . . .	1.8	1.8	1.7
Less developed regions . . .	4.2	3.8	3.5
Least developed countries . .	6.4	6.0	5.8
Africa	6.3	6.1	5.8
Eastern Africa	6.9	6.7	6.5
Middle Africa	6.5	6.5	6.5
Northern Africa	5.6	4.9	4.2
Southern Africa	4.9	4.5	4.2
Western Africa	6.7	6.6	6.5
Asia	3.7	3.4	3.0
Eastern Asia	2.4	2.3	1.9
South-central Asia	5.0	4.5	4.1
South-eastern Asia	4.2	3.7	3.3
Western Asia	5.0	4.7	4.4
Europe	1.9	1.8	1.6
Eastern Europe	2.1	2.1	1.6
Northern Europe	1.8	1.8	1.8
Southern Europe	1.8	1.6	1.4
Western Europe	1.6	1.6	1.5
Latin America	3.8	3.4	3.1
Caribbean	3.1	2.9	2.8
Central America	4.6	4.0	3.5
South America	3.7	3.2	3.0
Northern America	1.8	1.9	2.1
Oceania	2.6	2.6	2.5
Australia-New Zealand . . .	1.9	1.9	1.9

Source: World Population Prospects: The 1994 Revision (United Nations publication, Sales No. E.95.XIII.16), annex tables A.18 and A.19.
[a]Estimates for 1990-1995 are assumptions for the medium-variant projections.
[b]Number of births per woman.

Although adolescent fertility is increasingly perceived as an issue of social and policy concern, fertility rates among women under age 20 have been falling alongside overall fertility rates worldwide, owing to rising age at marriage, increasing educational opportunities for young women and increased use of contraception. There are, however, some exceptions to the overall downward trend—for example, in Haiti, India and the United States of America.

Education has long been recognized as a crucial factor influencing reproductive behaviour. According to a recent United Nations study, female education is universally associated with lower fertility (United Nations, 1995c). Countries in Latin America display the largest fertility gaps between better educated and uneducated women, ranging from three to five children per woman. Fertility differentials by education are not uniform across countries, suggesting that the resultant effect of women's education is conditioned by socio-economic development, social structure and cultural context. In contemporary developing societies, the impact of individual schooling on child-bearing tends to become stronger as the socio-economic conditions and the overall educational level of the society improve.

The direct and indirect paths through which female education influences reproductive behaviour are numerous. Education is associated with later entry into marriage, preferences for smaller families and increased awareness, acceptability and use of contraception. Unwanted or unplanned fertility is also lowest among better educated women, suggesting that education enables reproductive choice and enhances women's control over the process of family formation.

The timing of the onset of child-bearing has important implications for individuals, families and societies. In most countries, a woman's first child is born within one or two years after first marriage. However, marriage is not the only context within which child-bearing takes place. In many developed countries, the rapid increase in child-bearing outside marriage, closely linked to the rise in cohabitation, has been a significant social development during the past decade. In the developing regions, out-of-wedlock child-bearing is relatively rare in Asia, but commonplace in Africa and Latin America and the Caribbean, reflecting the high prevalence of consensual unions.

The timing of entry into motherhood is remarkably similar across a wide range of developing countries: it tends to occur between ages 19 and 22. In most developed countries, entry into motherhood occurs at a later age, usually between ages 22 and 27. The trend observed during the past decade in both developing and developed societies has been towards a delayed pattern of child-bearing. The span of women's child-bearing—that is, the average number of years between women's first and last birth—is longest in Africa (15-20 years), followed by Asia (11-17 years) and Latin America and the Caribbean (11-16 years).

Reproductive preferences play a crucial role in shaping the process of child-bearing. The number of children a woman desires not only depends upon her personal circumstances but is also conditioned by the socio-economic context, cultural values, family system and gender relations in the society where she lives. The current comprehensive approach to reproductive health has contributed to a redefining of the goals of family planning programmes, from an implicit concern with

14

reducing fertility to an explicit concern with assisting individuals to achieve their reproductive aspirations.

Fertility preferences vary considerably across regions. Desired family size is largest in sub-Saharan Africa (4-8 children), followed by Asia (3-5), Northern Africa, and Latin America and the Caribbean (3-4). The observed trend points towards women's increasing preference for smaller families.

The prevailing gap between women's ideal family size and actual child-bearing suggests that women's reproductive aspirations are seldom fulfilled. The inadequate control women have over their reproduction is also evident from the high prevalence of unplanned child-bearing. The percentage of births reportedly unwanted ranges from 2 to 26 in Africa, 6 to 21 in Asia and 5 to 35 in Latin America and the Caribbean, and the percentage of births reportedly mistimed ranges from 6 to 52 in Africa, 8 to 28 in Asia and 13 to 25 in Latin America and the Caribbean.

In the developed countries, a family with two children is the dominant ideal, and in many cases, the preferred number of children is above the actual total fertility rate. However, the number of unintended births is relatively large, despite the high prevalence of contraceptive use. In the United States, for example, 12 per cent of all births were reported as unwanted and 27 per cent as mistimed.

Since reproductive choice is seriously hampered in the presence of infertility, its prevention, diagnosis and treatment are increasingly recognized as a key component of reproductive health. Between 8 and 12 per cent of all couples experience some form of infertility during their reproductive life, a problem affecting from 50 million to 80 million people worldwide (WHO, 1991). In a small proportion of couples (under 5 per cent) the underlying causes of infertility are attributable to anatomical, genetic, endocrinological or immunological factors. However, in the majority of cases, problems of infertility arise from preventable causes, such as untreated infection from sexually transmitted disease, post-partum and post-abortion complications, or female genital mutilation.

Past studies have documented an unusually high incidence of impaired fertility in Africa, particularly in Central Africa. Recent DHS data show that, with regard to primary infertility (the inability to conceive or bear any children at all), the proportion of childless women among ever-married women aged 40-44 does not exceed 6 per cent in any of the surveyed countries. However, when secondary infertility (the inability to conceive or bear a child subsequent to an earlier birth) is examined, the prevalence of disease-induced sterility is significant: among women aged 30-34, the proportion is estimated to be above 20 per cent in Benin, Botswana, Côte d'Ivoire, Ghana, Liberia, Mali,

15

Figure II. Percentage of women receiving prenatal care and professional assistance at delivery

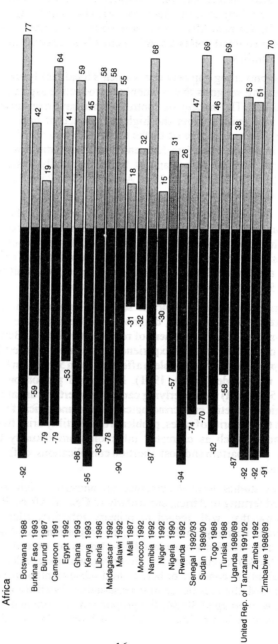

Africa

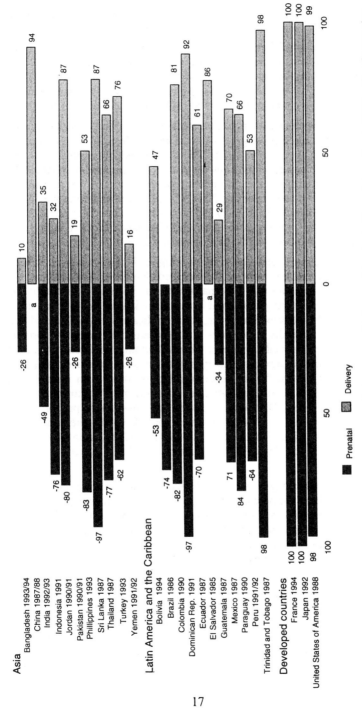

Asia

	Prenatal	Delivery
Bangladesh 1993/94	-26	10
China 1987/88	-49	94
India 1992/93	a	35
Indonesia 1991	-76	32
Jordan 1990/91	-80	87
Pakistan 1990/91	-26	19
Phillippines 1993	-83	53
Sri Lanka 1987	-97	87
Thailand 1987	-77	66
Turkey 1993	-62	76
Yemen 1991/92	-26	16

Latin America and the Caribbean

	Prenatal	Delivery
Bolivia 1994	-53	47
Brazil 1986	-74	81
Colombia 1990	-82	92
Dominican Rep. 1991	-97	61
Ecuador 1987	-70	86
El Salvador 1985	-34	29
Guatemala 1987	a	
Mexico 1987	71	70
Paraguay 1990	84	66
Peru 1991/92	-64	53
Trinidad and Tobago 1987	98	98

Developed countries

	Prenatal	Delivery
France 1994	100	100
Japan 1992	100	100
United States of America 1988	98	99

Prenatal ■   Delivery ▨

Sources: Dara Carr and Ann Way, *Women's Lives and Experiences* (Calverton, Maryland: Macro International, 1994); Alan Guttmacher Institute, *Hope and Realities* (New York, 1995).

NOTE: Based on births during the five years preceding the survey.

[a]Data not available on prenatal care.

17

Mauritania, Nigeria, Senegal, the Sudan, Uganda and Zimbabwe and above 30 per cent in Cameroon (Larsen, 1994).

A number of factors associated with the pattern of child-bearing may adversely affect the survival and well-being of mothers and children. Pregnancies too early or too late in the maternal life course, high-parity pregnancies and closely spaced pregnancies are considered to pose higher-than-normal risks to children's and women's health.

It has been documented that mother's age affects pregnancy outcomes, children's subsequent survival and the likelihood of complications during pregnancy and childbirth. Reproductive morbidity and mortality are more common among women who become pregnant at the very beginning and at the end of their reproductive span. The percentage of births to women under age 20 is 9 in the developed countries, 11 in the developing countries and 17 in the least developed countries. With regard to the prevalence of late child-bearing, Africa displays the highest proportion of births to women over age 34 (15 per cent).

The relation between birth-spacing and child survival is well established and extensively documented. However, the relation between birth-spacing and maternal health has been less systematically studied. Because pregnancy and lactation are known to put extra stress on women's nutritional reserves, some studies have hypothesized that short birth intervals, especially if accompanied by intensive breast-feeding, may prevent a woman from rebuilding depleted nutritional stores before the next pregnancy begins, in what is called "maternal depletion syndrome". The negative effect of short birth intervals on maternal health is largely contingent upon a woman's prior nutritional and health status. DHS data show that a considerable proportion of births are spaced less than two years apart from the previous birth, ranging from 10 to 29 per cent in sub-Saharan Africa, from 14 to 41 per cent in Asia and from 20 to 29 per cent in Latin America and the Caribbean.

Although changes in the age, parity and birth-spacing distributions of fertility have the potential of reducing maternal mortality, the majority of women who die from pregnancy, abortion or childbirth do not fall within those high-risk categories. Socio-economic conditions, education, nutrition and health care are often more important determinants of women's health and survival.

The risks associated with pregnancy and child-bearing can be substantially reduced through adequate obstetric and maternal care. Hence, the availability and quality of health-care services and access to them largely condition the impact of physiological risk factors on women's health. Coverage of maternity services varies greatly between countries. Data on the percentages of women receiving prenatal care and professional assistance in 46 developing and 3 developed countries are shown in figure II. In 15 out of 44 developing countries, the proportion of births for which women received prenatal care was below two thirds; in 17 out of 45 countries, fewer than 50 per cent of the deliveries were assisted by a trained professional.

III. CONTRACEPTION

Family planning is an integral part of reproductive health. Since the 1960s there has been a sustained increase in the use of contraception in developing countries. In the early 1960s, when TFR in the less developed regions averaged 6.1 children per woman, the level of contraceptive prevalence—-current use among couples with the woman of reproductive age—was probably under 10 per cent in the developing countries. Recent surveys show that contraceptive prevalence in those regions had risen to 53 per cent by 1991. In developed countries, contraceptive prevalence averaged 71 per cent, and for the world as a whole the average was 57 per cent (see table 5). The level of contraceptive use in Africa, at 19 per cent, is far below the average level for the other developing regions: 79 per cent in Eastern Asia; 43 per cent in the remainder of Asia and Oceania; and 59 per cent in Latin America and the Caribbean.

The transformation in contraceptive practice reflects the growing desire of couples and individuals to have smaller families and to choose when to have their children. It also reflects great increases in the availability of effective modern contraceptives in developing countries and of associated family planning information and services. Although the recent changes in the developed regions concern primarily the choice of specific birth control methods rather than the overall level of contraceptive use, the introduction of modern methods has also brought about a transformation in contraceptive practice.

Most users of contraception are women, and most of them use modern methods. Relatively effective clinic and supply ("modern") methods account for an estimated 87 per cent of contraceptive use worldwide. The three main "female" methods—female sterilization, intra-uterine devices (IUDs) and oral pills—account for over two thirds of contraceptive practice worldwide, and three fourths of use in the less developed regions. Modern methods in general make up a larger fraction of contraceptive use in the developing than in the developed countries, estimated at 91 and 73 per cent, respectively. Prevalence of clinic and supply methods averages 51 per cent in the more developed regions and 48 per cent in the less developed regions.

The prevalence of non-supply and traditional methods differs more between the developed and the developing countries: 20 and 5 per cent, respectively. This group of methods includes periodic abstinence or rhythm, withdrawal (coitus interruptus), abstinence, douching and various folk methods. The higher levels of use of these methods in the

20

TABLE 5. AVERAGE PREVALENCE OF SPECIFIC CONTRACEPTIVE METHODS, BY REGION[a]

(Percentage of couples with the woman of reproductive age)

Major area and region	All methods (1)	Modern methods[b] (2)	Sterilization Female (3)	Sterilization Male (4)	Pill (5)	Inject-able (6)	IUD (7)	Condom (8)	Vaginal barrier methods (9)	Rhythm (10)	With-drawal (11)	Other methods (12)
World	57	49	18	4	8	1	12	5	1	3	4	1
Less developed regions	53	48	21	4	6	2	13	2	0.2	2	2	1
Africa	19	15	1	0.1	7	2	4	1	0.2	2	1	1
Asia and Oceania[c]	58	54	24	5	5	2	16	2	0.2	2	2	0.3
Eastern Asia	79	79	33	9	3	0.1	31	2	0.3	0.4	0.1	..
Other countries	43	36	17	2	6	3	5	3	0.1	3	3	1
Latin America and the Carribean	59	49	21	1	17	1	6	2	1	6	3	0.5
More developed regions[d]	71	51	8	5	17	0.1	5	14	2	6	12	1

Source: World Population Monitoring, 1996 (United Nations publication, forthcoming).
NOTE: These estimates reflect assumptions about contraceptive use in countries with no available data.
[a]Based on the most recently available survey data: average date, 1991.
[b]Including methods in columns 3-9.
[c]Excluding Japan.
[d]Australia-New Zealand, Europe, Northern America and Japan.

developed countries reflects the continuing influence of patterns of fertility control established before the era of modern contraceptive methods and also the lack of wide availability of newer methods in some countries. Some developed countries in which the use of traditional methods was widespread around 1970 have undergone a marked transition to the use of modern methods: Belgium, France and Hungary are examples. However, some countries in Eastern Europe, based on surveys conducted in the 1990s, still show high prevalence levels of traditional methods; examples include the Czech Republic, Romania and Slovakia.

Most developing countries with available trend data show a substantial recent increase in contraceptive use. A consideration of trends between the most recent available survey and surveys conducted about 10 years earlier shows that increases in contraceptive use have been the most rapid in countries that had a moderate level of use at the beginning of the period. Where prevalence was in the range of 15-50 per cent, the level of contraceptive use subsequently grew by more than 1.0 percentage point per annum in over 80 per cent of the countries. By contrast, increases of that size or more occurred in only about 55 per cent of the countries where prevalence was initially either below 15 per cent or above 50 per cent. Although the average level of contraceptive use remains much lower in Africa than in other developing regions, surveys conducted in the past few years have continued to add to the evidence of increasing use of contraception in continental sub-Saharan Africa.

With respect to the use of particular types of contraception, rising use of female sterilization is the most important trend in both developed and developing countries. None the less, there are many individual countries where other methods are responsible for most of the recent trend. While there is a general tendency for modern methods as a group to become more predominant over time, there is little sign that the widely varying national patterns of use are converging to the same method mix. Only rarely does a single type of contraception account for most of current use.

Recent surveys indicate a significant rise in the level of use of condoms in several countries, suggesting that campaigns promoting this method are having an effect. On average, condoms account for only about 8 per cent of contraceptive practice reported by married women. However, men tend to report more use of this method than do women. Levels of condom use among unmarried men are usually higher than among married men, even though the general level of contraceptive use is higher among the married men.

Despite the recent rapid growth in the use of contraception, a variety of indicators suggest that the level of unmet need remains high: about 20-25 per cent of couples in developing countries (except China) are at risk of an unwanted or mistimed pregnancy but are not using

22

contraception. In Africa and in some countries in other regions, substantial proportions of the population still have no knowledge of any type of contraception. Furthermore, the percentage of women with knowledge of a place that provides family planning information or services is sometimes much lower than the percentage of those that have heard of a method. In Asia and Northern Africa, 90 per cent or more of women knew of a service outlet in over three fourths of the countries with available data, and in Latin America and the Caribbean this level was reached in about 60 per cent of countries. However, this level of knowledge of services was observed in only 2 of 23 countries in sub-Saharan Africa (Botswana and Zimbabwe).

In general, problems of limited knowledge of and access to family planning reflect the difficulty many Governments have experienced in extending services nationwide rather than a deliberate policy to restrict access. By 1995, only two Governments (out of 190) had an official policy of limiting access to modern contraceptive methods, while 82 per cent of the Governments provided direct support for family planning services. Ratings of various aspects of family planning policy and programme performance, carried out in 1982, 1989 and 1994, indicate that there was rapid growth in programme effort and method availability during the 1980s. A further increase was noted in many countries after 1989, but at a slower pace than between 1982 and 1989. Based on knowledgeable observers' ratings of the availability of five types of contraception, in 1994 condoms were estimated to be readily available to about two thirds of the population of developing countries, and oral pills, IUDs and female sterilization to about 60-65 per cent. Male sterilization was judged to be readily available to slightly less than 50 per cent of the population. Despite substantial recent improvements, contraceptive methods are much less readily available in sub-Saharan Africa than in other regions.

In most developing countries levels of contraceptive use are substantially higher among urban and well-educated women than among their rural and less educated counterparts. During the past 10-15 years, the average size of the social differentials in contraceptive practice has changed very little, although this is partially due to offsetting changes in different countries. Where contraceptive use had been low to start with, differentials usually widened, and the reverse was true in countries where use levels were already high at the earlier date in urban areas or among highly educated women.

Many surveys have limited questions about current contraceptive use to married women exclusively. Recently, more surveys have posed such questions to unmarried women, and the resultant data show that an exclusive focus on married women leaves out a significant proportion of contraceptive users in many cases. In sub-Saharan Africa and in the more developed regions with such information available, women not in a union make up about 25 per cent of all contraceptive users, on average, and in Latin America and the Caribbean, nearly 10 per cent.

While some couples use a single contraceptive method success-fully for many years, most are likely to stop contraceptive use or switch from their first method at some point. Studies of contraceptive discon-tinuation show that within a year of beginning to use the pill, typically 40-60 per cent of women will have stopped the use; IUD, 15-30 per cent; the condom, more than 50 per cent; and periodic abstinence (including the calendar rhythm method), about 40-60 per cent. Reasons for stopping vary by method. In general, methods that are highly effective at preventing pregnancy have a high incidence of side-effects, and vice versa.

Side-effects and worries about them stand out consistently in studies of different populations as one of women's major concerns about modern contraceptive methods. Health concerns and side-effects are frequently cited as the reason for discontinuing a method, and in many cases a substantial proportion of women who are at risk of an unwanted pregnancy report that health concerns are their main reason for not using contraception. At the same time, the recent rise in the level of contraceptive use is due almost entirely to increased use of modern methods. The evidence thus suggests that, although modern methods have worked well for many couples, their use still presents difficult choices for many others. The rapidly increasing reliance on the perma-nent method of surgical sterilization must in part reflect the drawbacks of the temporary methods and services that are currently available.

Although most information about contraceptive use and unmet need is derived from surveys of women, recently more surveys have asked men about these topics. This information is only now beginning to be analysed in detail. In some countries a substantial proportion of the women with an apparent unmet need for contraception report that they are not using any method because of opposition from their spouse, which could refer either to opposition to contraception in general or to a disagreement about the number and timing of children. The available evidence about disagreements between spouses points to a variety of situations whose relative importance is often impossible to quantify. Some men clearly do expect to make the choice about using contracep-tion (even if it is the woman that uses the method), while others view this as being completely the woman's responsibility. In some countries, many people do not know their partner's views about family planning. The question of how inter-spouse disagreements are resolved in practice deserves more attention than it has received to date, and this requires obtaining comparable information from both men and women.

IV. ABORTION

Approximately 25 million legal abortions were performed world-wide around 1990, or one legal abortion for every six births. This estimate must be considered the minimum number, as no attempt has been made to estimate the magnitude of unreported legal abortions. In addition, WHO has estimated that some 20 million unsafe abortions are performed each year, or one unsafe abortion for every seven births (WHO, 1994).

Induced abortion has attained high public visibility in many countries, both developed and developing. In some cases, public concern has been voiced primarily because of the alarmingly high levels of maternal mortality and morbidity that have resulted from unsafe abortion. In others, the visibility has resulted more from public debate concerning the moral and legal status of abortion and the role that the State should play in permitting or denying access to safe abortion.

At the International Conference on Population and Development in 1994, the issue of abortion proved to be one of the most contentious, with much of the debate dealing directly or indirectly with various abortion-related issues. At the end of the debate, delegations agreed on the following text:

"In no case should abortion be promoted as a method of family planning. All Governments and relevant intergovernmental and non-governmental organizations are urged to strengthen their commitment to women's health, to deal with the health impact of unsafe abortion[2] as a major public health concern and to reduce the recourse to abortion through expanded and improved family-planning services. Prevention of unwanted pregnancies must always be given the highest priority and every attempt should be made to eliminate the need for abortion. Women who have unwanted pregnancies should have ready access to reliable information and compassionate counselling. Any measures or changes related to abortion within the health system can only be determined at the national or local level according to the national legislative process. In circumstances where abortion is not against the law, such abortion should be safe. In all cases, women should have access to quality services for the management of complications arising from abortion. Post-abortion counselling, education and family-planning services should be offered promptly, which will also help to avoid repeat abortions." (United Nations, 1995a, chap. I, resolution 1, annex, para. 8.25)

In the light of this recommendation, at the Fourth World Conference on Women, held at Beijing in September 1995, Governments were urged to consider reviewing laws containing punitive measures against women who have undergone illegal abortions.

Induced abortion is one of the oldest methods of fertility control and one of the most widely used (United Nations, 1992, 1993 and 1995d). It is practised both in remote rural societies and in large modern urban centres and in all regions of the world, although with differing consequences. When performed by appropriately qualified practitioners under hygienic circumstances, induced abortions generally pose a relatively small threat to women's reproductive health. Where abortion is illegal, however, it is usually performed in medically substandard and unsanitary conditions, leading to a high incidence of complications and resulting in chronic morbidity and often death. Indeed, WHO has estimated that approximately 76,000 women die annually as a result of complications arising from unsafe abortion. Moreover, long-term consequences of unsafe abortion may include chronic pelvic pain, pelvic inflammatory disease, tubal occlusion, secondary infertility and increased risk of spontaneous abortion in subsequent pregnancies (WHO, 1994).

Substantial variations exist in the incidence of unsafe abortion by region, from a high of 30 or more per 1,000 women aged 15-49 years in Eastern and Western Africa, Latin America and the Caribbean and the former Union of Soviet Socialist Republics, to a negligible number in Northern Europe and Northern America (WHO, 1994). Some of the variations can be explained by the less restrictive nature of abortion laws in Northern Europe and Northern America, where 11 of 12 countries permit abortion on request or for economic or social reasons, as compared with those in Eastern and Western Africa and Latin America and the Caribbean, where 2 of 45 countries permit abortion on request or for economic or social reasons. Lack of legal restrictions on abortion, however, does not necessarily guarantee access to safe abortion, as evidenced by the relatively high incidence of unsafe abortion in the former USSR (estimated by WHO at 30 unsafe abortions per 1,000 women aged 15-49 years), despite the availability of abortion on request since 1956.

In line with the heightened interest in adolescent reproductive behaviour, adolescent abortion is a growing area of concern. Because adolescents are sometimes unwilling or unable to seek appropriate health care or because they may wait longer in the gestation period to obtain help, induced abortion generally presents a greater risk to the health and life of an adolescent than to an adult woman. According to recent United Nations estimates, abortion among adolescents has accounted for 15-25 per cent of total reported legal abortions in a number of developed and developing countries.

Based on information available for 193 countries, the overwhelming majority of countries (98 per cent) permit abortions to be performed to save the pregnant woman's life (see figure III; and United Nations,

26

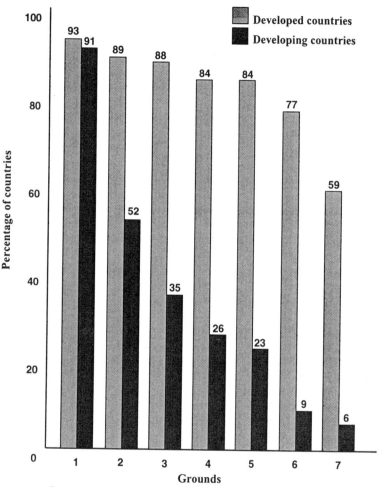

Grounds:
1. To save the life of the woman
2. To preserve physical health
3. To preserve mental health
4. Rape or incest
5. Foetal impairment
6. Economic or social reasons
7. Available on request

Sources: *Abortion Policies: A Global Review*, vol. I, *Afghanistan to France* (United Nations publication, Sales No. E.92.XIII.3); vol. II, *Gabon to Norway* (United Nations publication, Sales No. E.94.XIII.2);vol. III, *Oman to Zimbabwe* (United Nations publication, Sales No. E.95.XIII.24).

1992, 1993 and 1995d). In a number of those countries, criminal law specifically allows abortion on this ground. In others, however, one must look to other laws or court decisions to determine whether there are exceptions to a general prohibition of abortion. For example, in Honduras, the Code of Medical Ethics permits abortion to save the woman's life; in Nepal, the rules of the Medical Council have been interpreted to permit abortion in various situations; and in Ireland the Supreme Court has ruled that an abortion can be performed to preserve the life of the pregnant woman. In yet other countries, such as the Central African Republic, the Dominican Republic, Egypt and the Philippines, the criminal law principle of necessity can be invoked to exempt from punishment the performance of an abortion to save a pregnant woman's life.

Abortion to preserve the woman's physical health is permitted in 119 countries (62 per cent). Fewer countries (95, or 50 per cent) allow abortion to preserve the woman's mental health, and 81 countries (42 per cent) permit it when pregnancy has resulted from rape or incest. The number declines to 78 countries (40 per cent) when there is the possibility of foetal impairment and to 55 countries (29 per cent) when the reasons are economic or social. Lastly, in 41 countries (21 per cent), abortion is available on request.

An examination of abortion policies in terms of population discloses that 96 per cent of the world population live in countries that permit abortion to save the woman's life, 75 per cent live in countries permitting abortion to preserve the woman's physical health, 69 per cent in countries where abortion is legal to preserve the woman's mental health and 72 per cent in countries where abortion is allowed when the pregnancy results from rape or incest. The percentage declines to 64 when there is the possibility of foetal impairment and to 44 in countries that permit abortion for economic or social reasons. Lastly, abortion is available on request to 38 per cent of the world population.

V. MATERNAL MORTALITY AND MORBIDITY

Among the health and mortality indicators, levels of maternal mortality show striking disparities according to level of development. Maternal mortality is a sensitive indicator of the status of women in society, their access to health care and the adequacy of the health care system in responding to their needs. Information about levels and trends of maternal mortality is needed, therefore, not only for assessing the risks of pregnancy and childbirth, but also for determining what maternal mortality implies about the health of women in general and, by extension, about their social and economic well-being.

It is extremely difficult to assess levels of maternal mortality at the national level. Doing so requires knowledge about deaths of women of reproductive age (15-49 years), the cause of death and also whether or not the woman was pregnant at the time of death or had recently been so. Few countries register all births and deaths; even fewer register the cause of death; and fewer still systematically note pregnancy status on the death form.

Inevitably, countries with the least developed systems of vital registration are those with the worst health indicators. In such circumstances, alternative ways have to be developed for estimating levels of maternal mortality. A variety of innovative methodologies has been devised to overcome the absence of data in countries with poor or non-existent vital registration. For example, maternal mortality can be measured by incorporating questions on pregnancy and death into large-scale household inquiries, but this approach requires a large sample size and is expensive and time-consuming. A more cost-effective approach is the "sisterhood method", which adds on to existing household surveys a few simple questions about whether or not the sisters of the respondent are still alive. Much smaller sample sizes are needed because each respondent can provide information on a number of sisters. However, the results do not provide current estimates but only give an idea of the levels of maternal mortality roughly 10 years earlier.

The best way to measure maternal mortality in the absence of vital registration is to identify and investigate the causes of all deaths of women of reproductive age—the Reproductive Age Mortality Survey (RAMOS). Multiple sources of information—civil registers, health facility records, community leaders, religious authorities, undertakers, cemetery officials, schoolchildren—must be used to identify all deaths. Subsequently, health-care providers, facility records and interviews with household members are used to classify deaths as maternal or otherwise (verbal autopsy). Although RAMOS studies are considered to be the best method for estimating maternal mortality, they are time-consuming and complex to undertake, particularly on a large scale.

Because of the difficulties and costs involved, only 10 developing countries have carried out RAMOS or household studies at the national level. As a result, other methods have to be devised to provide broad estimates of the extent of the problem. WHO and the United Nations Children's Fund (UNICEF) have developed a new approach for estimating maternal mortality and recently issued new data at the national, regional and international levels. The new estimates were developed using a dual strategy: existing national maternal mortality estimates were adjusted to account for underreporting and misclassification, and a simple model was developed to predict values for countries with no data. The model uses two independent variables—general fertility rates and proportion of births that are assisted by a trained person—to predict maternal mortality.

The new approach is primarily intended to be useful in countries with no estimates of maternal mortality or where there is concern about the adequacy of officially reported estimates. The intention was to draw attention to the existence and likely dimensions of the problem of maternal mortality. The estimates should be taken as indicating orders of magnitude rather than precise estimates and are not necessarily those considered by Governments as the most appropriate. The results for each country should serve as a stimulus to action and to help mobilize national and external resources to that end. The standard errors associated with the predicted maternal mortality ratios are very large. They cannot, therefore, be used to monitor trends on a year-to-year basis but may be used to monitor changes over the decade. The figures pertain to 1990 and should be seen as a recalculation of the 1991 revision rather than as indicative of trends since then.

Results of the new model, shown in table 6, indicate that maternal mortality is higher than previously estimated, with some 585,000 maternal deaths in 1990, compared with 509,000, according to the earlier model. The most significant differences between the old and the new models are for Africa, where the maternal mortality ratio according to the new estimates is 870 per 100,000 live births, compared with the earlier estimate of 630 per 100,000. By contrast, the estimates produced by the new model for Asia and Latin America and the Caribbean show relatively little change compared with the earlier model.

If counting the total numbers of maternal deaths is difficult, estimating the causes of those deaths is even more so. Few studies collect information on the cause of death in a standard format or follow the categories of causes of death described in the International Classification of Diseases. However, based on the evidence of the few good

TABLE 6.   ESTIMATES OF MATERNAL DEATHS AND MATERNAL
MORTALITY RATIOS, BY MAJOR AREA AND REGION, 1990

Major area and region	Maternal deaths	
	Number (thousands)	Ratio (per 100,000 live births)
World	85	30
More developed regions[a]	4	27
Less developed regions[b]	582	480
Africa	235	870
Asia	325	380
Europe	3.2	36
Latin America and the Caribbean . . .	23	190
Northern America	0.5	11
Oceania	1.4	380

Source: World Health Organization, "New estimates of maternal mortality",
Weekly Epidemiological Record (Geneva), vol. 71, No. 13 (1996), pp. 97-100.
[a]More developed regions comprise all regions in Europe, Northern America
and Australia, New Zealand and Japan.
[b]Less developed regions comprise all regions of Africa, Asia (excluding Japan),
Latin America and the Caribbean and regions of Melanesia, Micronesia and Polynesia.

community-based studies, it is possible to estimate the breakdown of
maternal mortality by five major causes of death. A summary of the
incidence of and mortality from the five major obstetric complications
is given in table 7. There are significant regional variations within these
global totals. Abortion is likely to account for a larger percentage
of overall maternal mortality in Latin America and the Caribbean,
although the maternal mortality ratio is generally lower in that region
than in most parts of Africa.

In these calculations it has been assumed that each complication
is a discrete event and that, therefore, complications arise in some
56 per cent of pregnancies ending in live birth. The severity of the
complication will, of course, vary, and WHO estimates that almost
15 per cent of all women develop complications serious enough to
require rapid and skilled intervention if the woman is to survive without
lifelong disabilities. Such disabilities include obstetric fistula (damage
to the bladder and/or rectum); reproductive tract infections; pelvic
inflammatory disease; infertility; anaemia; prolapse; and damage to the
brain, kidneys and cardiovascular system.

The complications that cause the deaths and disabilities of mothers
also damage the infants they are carrying (see table 8). Of the approximately 8 million infant deaths each year, almost two thirds occur during
the neonatal period, before the baby is one month old. Of the 5 million
neonatal deaths, 3.5 million occur within the first week of life and are

31

TABLE 7. ESTIMATED GLOBAL INCIDENCE OF AND MORTALITY FROM MAIN OBSTETRIC COMPLICATIONS WORLDWIDE, 1990

Obstetric complication	Number of cases[a] (thousands)	Number of deaths (thousands)	Percentage of all maternal deaths
Haemorrhage	13 700	76	25
Sepsis	11 500	87	15
Hypertensive disorders of pregnancy and eclampsia	6 800	74	13
Obstructed labour	7 000	44	7
Unsafe abortion	19 400	76	13
Other direct causes	3 400	44	8
Indirect causes	13 000	115	19
Total	75 000	585	100

Source: World Health Organization, Maternal Health and Safe Motherhood Programme (Geneva), unpublished provisional estimates.
[a]Estimated number of events, not women.

TABLE 8. EFFECTS OF PREGNANCY COMPLICATIONS ON MOTHER AND BABY

Problem or compilation	Most serious effects on mother's health	Most serious effects on newborn baby
Severe anaemia	Cardiac failure	Low birth weight, asphyxia, stillbirth
Haemorrhage	Shock, cardiac failure, infection	Asphyxia, stillbirth
Hypertensive disorders of pregnancy	Eclampsia, cerebrovascular accidents	Low birth weight, asphyxia, stillbirth
Puerperal sepsis	Septicaemia, shock	Neonatal sepsis
Obstructed labour	Fistulae, uterine rupture, prolapse,amnionitis, sepsis	Stillbirth, asphyxia, sepsis, birth trauma, handicap
Infection during pregnancy, sexually transmitted diseases	Premature onset of labour, ectopic pregnancy, pelvic inflammatory disease, infertility	Premature delivery, neonatal eye infection, blindness, pneumonia, stillbirth, congenital syphilis
Hepatitis	Post-partum haemorrhage, liver failure	Hepatitis
Malaria	Severe anaemia, cerebral thrombosis	Prematurity, intra-uterine growth retardation
Unwanted pregnancy	Unsafe abortion, infection, pelvic inflammatory disease	Increased risk of morbidity and mortality
Unclean delivery	Infection, maternal tetanus	Neonatal tetanus, sepsis

largely a consequence of inadequate or inappropriate care during pregnancy, delivery or the first critical hours after birth. And for every newborn death, another infant is stillborn.

Aside from considerations of the number of deaths and disabilities, there is also the issue of the nature of maternal death. The mothers who die are in the prime of life, at the peak of their social and economic productivity. They leave behind their families, many with young children, that must survive without the support of the prime caregiver, producer of food and generator of income.

The paucity of information about maternal ill-health has resulted in long neglect of the problem, neglect that the international community has only recently started to address. There is still much that has to be learned, not about the interventions needed to reduce maternal deaths—which have been known for many years—but about how to implement those interventions in a sustainable way in resource-limited settings. Although maternal mortality and morbidity are major components of reproductive ill-health, addressing them requires interventions that differ, in several important ways, from the interventions needed to deal with other components of reproductive ill-health. In particular, it will not be possible to achieve sustainable reductions in maternal mortality in the absence of functioning district health systems, including widespread availability of maternal health care at the community level, along with appropriate referral and management of complications and emergencies.

VI. SEXUALLY TRANSMITTED DISEASES, INCLUDING HIV/AIDS

Until recently, the prevention and control of sexually transmitted diseases was given low priority by most countries and development agencies. Several factors have played a role in this respect: lack of awareness of the problem of sexually transmitted diseases and their complications and sequelae; competition for resources to control other important health problems; and reluctance of public health policy makers to deal with diseases associated with sexual behaviour.

To date, most programmes for the prevention of sexually transmitted diseases have focused on prevention of complications (secondary prevention). The prevention of the transmission of infection (primary prevention) is at present receiving increased attention because of the global HIV/AIDS epidemic and the identification of several sexually transmitted diseases as risk factors for the spread of HIV.

Currently in its second decade, the HIV epidemic continues to grow, with thousands of new infections occurring every day. An estimated cumulative total of 18.5 million adults (see table 9) and 1.5 million children have been infected with HIV. Of all the infected cases, from 7 million to 8 million are women, about 70 per cent of whom are of child-bearing age. According to WHO, between 13 million and 15 million infected adolescents and adults, in addition to about half a million infected children, are alive today.

The longer term dimensions of the HIV/AIDS pandemic cannot yet be forecast with confidence. However, on the basis of available data on the current global status of the pandemic and recent trends in its spread, WHO has generated a plausible range of projected new HIV infections during the 1990s. In making projections of the future magnitude of the pandemic, WHO uses the lower limit of its estimated range of the HIV prevalence for each region. The results should thus be considered conservative.

During the current decade, WHO forecasts that from about 10 million to 15 million new cases of HIV infections may be expected in adults, mostly in developing countries. During the same period, WHO projects that from as many as 5 million to 10 million children will be HIV-infected through their mothers, the majority of them in sub-Saharan Africa. By the year 2000, 30-40 million HIV infections will have occurred, 90 per cent of which will be in developing countries. The projected cumulative total number of HIV-related deaths is predicted to rise to more than 8 million from its current total of 2 million.

TABLE 9. ESTIMATED DISTRIBUTION OF CUMULATIVE HIV INFECTIONS IN ADULTS, BY MAJOR AREA AND REGION, MID-1995

Major area and region	Distribution
Africa	
Northern Africa/Western Asia	150 000+
Sub-Saharan Africa	11 000 000+
Asia	
Eastern Asia and the Pacific	50 000+
Southern/South-eastern Asia	3 500 000+
Australasia	25 000+
Europe	
Eastern Europe and Central Asia	50 000+
Western Europe	600 000+
Latin America and the Caribbean	2 000 000+
Northern America	1 100 000+

Source: World Health Organization. "The current global situation of the HIV/AIDS pandemic" (Geneva, 3 July 1995).

Table 10 shows estimates, by region, of the number of adults infected with HIV and alive as of mid-1994 and projections of the number of HIV-infected adults that will be living in the year 2000 (WHO, 1995a). WHO also estimates that over 5 million children under age 10 will be orphaned by the end of the 1990s as a result of the HIV-related deaths of their parents. The number of orphans will increase further in the early years of the twenty-first century as a result of the death of those mothers who were infected with HIV in the 1990s.

TABLE 10. ESTIMATED AND PROJECTED HIV PREVALENCE IN ADULTS, BY MAJOR AREA
(Millions)

Major area	Estimated HIV prevalence, mid-1994	Projected HIV prevalence, 2000
Australasia, Europe and Northern America . .	>1.2	1
Latin America and the Caribbean	>1.5	>2
Africa	>8	>9
Asia	>2.5	8
Global	13-14	>20

Source: World Health Organization, "The HIV/AIDS pandemic: 1994 overview" (Geneva, 1994), WHO/GPA/TCO/SEF/94.4.

35

The epidemic is having devastating effects on individuals, families and entire communities. For women, HIV infection has added its burden to risks related to sexually transmitted diseases, pregnancy and childbirth. The proportion of women with HIV and AIDS has increased, especially in developing countries. Young people are particularly affected by HIV and AIDS: it is estimated that 50 per cent of HIV infections occur in age group 15-24. This has an important impact on the economy of many countries since the age groups most affected—young and middle-aged adults—constitute the bulk of the workforce. The socio-economic burden of sexually transmitted diseases, in terms of direct and indirect costs, is increasing rapidly.

Over the past 10 years, the response to HIV/AIDS has focused on prevention and care. Governments, non-governmental organizations, communities, associations and networks of people living with HIV/AIDS, international organizations, the health, educational and other sectors, and the public and private sectors have worked in partnership to develop a response to the epidemic.

The epidemiological trends of sexually transmitted diseases in various parts of the world are strikingly different. In the developing countries the epidemic is characterized by high incidence and prevalence; a high rate of complication; an alarming problem of anti-microbial resistance; and the interaction with HIV infection. It is estimated that about 333 million curable cases of sexually transmitted diseases occur globally every year, most of them in developing countries (see table 11).

Sexually transmitted diseases have been a neglected area in public health in most of the developing countries, despite the overwhelming facts of their impact on health, particularly for women and newborns. For several decades, sexually transmitted diseases have ranked among the top five conditions for which adults in many developing countries seek health-care services. In most industrialized countries, on the other hand, there has been a spectacular decline in the incidence of sexually transmitted diseases, particularly gonorrhoea and syphilis.

Chlamydia infection is by far the most common bacterial sexually transmitted disease in Europe. For some time its incidence had been seriously underestimated because of a lack of diagnostic facilities. In countries with an active chlamydia control policy, there has been a well-documented reduction in the number of cases, particularly in women.

Reliable data on the incidence of sexually transmitted diseases in developing countries are scarce, although prevalence surveys have been conducted in many countries, particularly in Africa. In general, the survey data show higher rates of gonorrhoea, syphilis and chlamydia than in comparable populations in Europe or Northern America. How-

TABLE 11. NEW CASES OF CURABLE SEXUALLY TRANSMITTED DISEASES AMONG ADULTS, BY MAJOR AREA AND REGION, 1995

Major area and region	Number of cases (millions)
Africa	
Northern Africa/Western Asia	10
Sub-Saharan Africa	65
Asia	
Eastern Asia and the Pacific	23
Southern/South-eastern Asia	150
Australasia	1
Europe	
Eastern Europe and Central Asia	18
Western Europe	16
Latin America and the Caribbean	36
Northern America	14

Source: World Health Organization, *An Overview of Selected Curable Sexually Transmitted Diseases* (Geneva, 1995).

ever, there is also a large variation in prevalence, with some populations having low levels of infection. It should be stressed that the prevalence rate of a bacterial sexually transmitted disease is the result of both sexual exposure of the population and the proportion of infections adequately treated.

Women, especially young women, are more vulnerable than men to infection with a sexually transmitted disease and its complications (such as infertility, cancer and inflammatory diseases). The high prevalence of sexually transmitted diseases among women attending antenatal, family planning and gynaecological clinics in developing countries provides an indication of the extent of the problem. For example, in studies in developing countries, up to 19 per cent of the pregnant women have been found to have gonorrhoea or chlamydia, and up to 20 per cent to have syphilis.

Biologically women are more susceptible than men to most sexually transmitted diseases, at least in part because of the greater mucosal surface exposed to a greater quantity of pathogens during sexual intercourse. Women with a sexually transmitted disease are more likely than men to be asymptomatic and, therefore, are less likely to seek treatment, resulting in chronic infections with more long-term complications and sequelae.

There are important overlaps between programmes for the prevention of HIV/AIDS and sexually transmitted diseases and care programmes and other components of reproductive health programmes. Family planning services and maternal health/antenatal care services offer an important opportunity for both diagnosis and treatment of sexually transmitted diseases and information about their prevention, including safer sexual behaviour and related services such as the provision of condoms.

VII. REPRODUCTIVE RIGHTS

Reproductive health and reproductive rights are relatively new concepts in the area of population policy. They are also a particularly controversial topic. They relate to areas of life that are the most intimate and personal, such as sexuality, sexual relations and reproduction, as well as to matters that are central to how the members of a family relate to one another and how they perceive themselves. They are also linked with the status of women and the empowerment of women, matters which themselves provoke controversy in many countries.

Reproductive rights may be viewed as certain rights that all persons possess which will allow them access to the full range of reproductive health care. In particular, as formulated at the past three international conferences on population and at the Fourth World Conference on Women, these rights rest on the recognition of the basic right of all couples and individuals to decide freely and responsibly the number, spacing and timing of their children and to have the information and means to do so. They include the right to attain the highest standard of sexual and reproductive health and the right to make reproductive decisions free from discrimination, coercion and violence, as expressed in human rights documents. Furthermore, the Programme of Action of the International Conference on Population and Development and the Platform for Action of the Fourth World Conference on Women make clear that all of these rights are grounded in national laws, international human rights instruments and other international consensus documents.

Although the concept of reproductive rights is of relatively recent origin, there is ample support for those rights in existing international documents and human rights treaties. For example, the final documents adopted at all three international conferences on population and at the Fourth World Conference on Women, drawing upon the language originally formulated at the International Conference on Human Rights, held at Tehran in 1968, strongly support reproductive rights. Although the documents are not legally binding in terms of international law, they do bear great normative authority and have been endorsed by the vast majority of Governments.

Formal international treaties that are legally binding also support the concept of reproductive rights, if not by name. For example, the International Covenant on Civil and Political Rights contains a number of provisions that are relevant to the right to make voluntary decisions about bearing children.[3] Similarly, the International Covenant on Economic, Social and Cultural Rights recognizes the right of persons to enjoy the highest standards of health and calls for special attention to be given to women before and after childbirth and to the reduction of infant mortality.[3] With the approval of the Convention on the Elimination of All Forms of Discrimination against Women[4] in 1979, those reproductive rights are made explicit and strongly endorsed. National laws that support reproductive rights relating to maternal/child health care, access to the various forms of family planning, sex education and treatment and prevention of sexually transmitted diseases are common in both developing and developed countries.

One of the cornerstones of the concept of reproductive rights is the right of access to methods of family planning. This idea has been fundamental to definitions of reproductive rights from the beginning, appearing repeatedly in population and human rights documents as the right to have the "information and means" to decide freely and responsibly the number and spacing of children. Without such access, reproductive rights have, practically speaking, no real meaning.

Adolescent reproductive behaviour has become an emerging worldwide concern. Most countries do not have coherent policies for the protection and maintenance of reproductive health in adolescents, partly because of the sensitivity of the subject. Several key issues concerning the reproductive rights of adolescents pertain to marriage. In many parts of the world, women's basic human rights are violated when they are given in marriage without their consent. Moreover, despite legislation designed to eliminate the practice, girls in many countries marry shortly after puberty and are expected to start having children almost immediately, in part because of a lack of alternative opportunities. The adverse effects of early child-bearing are not only biomedical but also educational and economic, in the form of reduced opportunities for young mothers.

Many obstacles exist to the achievement of reproductive rights and reproductive health. Because of the sensitive and controversial character of the issues involved—in particular, sexuality, contraception, the empowerment of women and family relations—there is resistance to the expansion of reproductive rights. Another major problem is conceptual in nature. In many countries, human and reproductive rights, as expressed in international documents, are not familiar to the general public and little information is disseminated on them. In addition, human and reproductive rights may seem abstract in their formulation or even foreign to local experiences, attitudes and traditions. The less educated are especially likely to lack knowledge about their rights. Also, women more than men are subject to restrictions on their personal status which prevent them from obtaining information on their rights. Thus, many women are not aware that they have reproductive rights and are therefore unlikely to exercise them.

Action to achieve reproductive rights and health is restricted in scope by those obstacles. However, one strategy to overcome such obstacles is to try to strengthen and make greater use of international monitoring mechanisms. Another is to increase the provision of information and education on reproductive rights and reproductive health. Efforts can be increased to reach the millions of persons throughout the world who have little knowledge or understanding of reproductive health. These efforts cover basic facts on health and the reproductive system and the connection between reproductive health and such matters as age at marriage, level of education, the status of women and harmful practices, such as female genital mutilation. Greater publicity can also be given to the existence at the international level of the documents that countries have ratified which support rights on such matters, particularly the right to decide freely and responsibly the number and spacing of children. Moreover, to be effective, this information should be provided to medical personnel, religious leaders, government officials and non-governmental organizations.

The concept of reproductive rights must be presented in ways that are appropriate at the local level. One approach is to point to local laws that themselves support reproductive rights, such as the constitutions, population policies and health laws of various countries. Another is to draw on local social movements and traditions that support reproductive rights. A third approach is to relate "rights" language to actual needs at the local level—needs for basic health services, family planning and education, for example. If reproductive rights and reproductive health are to be secured at the local level, they need be integrated into existing societal structures and thus become part of the fabric of society.

VIII. POPULATION INFORMATION, EDUCATION AND COMMUNICATION

In the field of population, the phrase "information, education and communication" refers to the combination of all three processes in efforts to create public awareness of and advocacy for action on population and development issues. "Information, education and communication programme interventions" refers to that part of a country development programme which is directed to achieving measurable changes in the behaviour and attitude of specific audiences, based on a study of their needs and perceptions.

The implementation of the Programme of Action of the International Conference on Population and Development requires political support and advocacy, understood here as full commitment to its principles, goals and objectives. Effective advocacy is essential in creating awareness of reproductive rights and reproductive health and can be facilitated by the use of effective information, education and communication strategies. The importance of information, education and communication in the area of reproductive rights and reproductive health derives from the recognition that they are important instruments that stimulate attitudinal and behavioural change. In the area of human reproduction and health, various strategies have been used in attempts to develop positive attitudes and encourage responsible and healthy behaviour, help increase community participation in population activities and facilitate acceptance of population programmes in diverse cultural settings.

A primary aim of information, education and communication activities should be to motivate policy makers, programme managers, service providers and communities to translate into action the concept of reproductive rights and reproductive health, including family planning. This will require the strengthening of national capacities to undertake appropriate information, education and communication activities. It will also require that information, education and communication messages be effective and that service-delivery systems respond to the increased demand that those messages contribute to generating.

Information, education and communication programmes may combine strategies of mass, group and one-to-one communication approaches and use a variety of channels, from interpersonal and peer support to formal school curricula, from traditional and folk media to mass entertainment and news media, and production and dissemination of specific materials. The spectrum of activities includes awareness-raising campaigns; art exhibits and painting and poster competitions; design, development and distribution of information, education and communication and training materials; printing and distribution of booklets, brochures and comic books with family planning, sexual health and HIV/AIDS–prevention messages; radio and television programmes, particularly soap operas with family planning and HIV/AIDS themes; dramas and puppet shows; seminars and workshops; telephone hot lines; and preventive counselling, including the distribution of condoms. When planned in a coordinated and strategic manner, these activities can make a significant contribution to the impact of population programmes.

Three key issues have been identified in population information, education and communication programmes. First, social, cultural and political conditions can affect the recognition of reproductive rights and may limit access to reproductive health services and information; myths and ignorance may constitute major obstacles. Secondly, information, education and communication activities are not always properly linked to the delivery of reproductive health and family planning information and services. And thirdly, there is need for adequate indicators for measuring progress in this field.

Population policies and legislation have a major role to play in the creation of a supportive environment for reproductive health and family planning. Information, education and communication activities are facilitated when they are supported by population policies and appropriate legislation. It is also recognized that information, education and communication activities are valuable instruments for facilitating the understanding and acceptance of the goals and objectives of population policies.

Reproductive health and family planning programmes are usually a major component of national population policies and strategies, and information, education and communication activities provide strong programme support. Strengthening their links will make them mutually supportive and thus enable national programmes to better satisfy unmet demands through the delivery of high-quality reproductive health and family planning services. Many of the programmes include the prevention and control of sexually transmitted diseases and HIV/AIDS, and information, education and communication activities that are valuable tools in reaching groups at risk, especially adolescents, and in raising awareness and promoting behavioural change.

Population education is another common strategy adopted by Governments as part of their population policies. It usually covers such topics as population dynamics, pregnancy and family planning, family life, sex education and, more recently, new ways of looking at gender issues, and HIV/AIDS and sexually transmitted diseases. There is increasing evidence that sex and HIV/AIDS education programmes may reduce unsafe practices among sexually active adolescents and reduce early pregnancies.

The Programme of Action of the International Conference on Population and Development calls for a coordinated strategic approach to information, education and communication, which should be linked to, and complement, national population and development policies and strategies and a full range of services in reproductive health, including family planning and sexual health. Achieving such an objective requires that special attention be given to the following priority areas:

(*a*) *Data requirements, indicators and future research.* The development of appropriate mechanisms for collecting data and of instruments for assessing and evaluating programme results should receive high priority. Assistance to country programmes for developing or strengthening their information systems for the management of information, education and communication programmes should be a priority;

(*b*) *Adolescents.* Because of the critical stage of their personal development, young people, particularly adolescents, have special need for information on sexual and reproductive health, and on such related issues as substance abuse and violence. Providing information on sexuality, pregnancy and sexually transmitted diseases, combined with information about local services and counselling availability, is an effective way of assisting them. Their participation in such activities can help ensure that the messages are appropriate and compelling to their peers. They can also be involved in facilitating the community dialogue and debate that should be linked to those efforts. Youth organizations can also play a major role in health promotion for youth, both in and out of school, and contribute to making young people's immediate environment more supportive. Youth groups can make linkages with the health sector and help make health services more "youth friendly". Such organizations can also play a role in involving parents and helping them understand and provide support to their adolescent children;

(*c*) *Gender equality and equity.* The Programme of Action affirms that the full participation and partnership of both women and men is required in reproductive life. Education and information that promote such aims, along with responsible sexuality and respect for women, are also fundamental to improving the status and role of women in society. Increasing the education given to girls and women contributes to their empowerment and to improved family health. Expanding women's knowledge of reproductive health and expanding their choices enables them to meet their reproductive goals. Information, education and communication activities can contribute to eradicating harmful practices against women and girls, such as female genital mutilation; drawing attention to the health needs of the girl-child; eliminating nutrition practices that discriminate against girls; involving men in reproductive health and family planning programmes; removing barriers to women's rights and enforcing legislation on early marriage, sexual exploitation and violence; and ensuring that women have equal access to education, are guaranteed equal opportunity to work and receive equal pay for equal work;

(d) *Participation of programme users.* The participation of programme users in the design, implementation and evaluation of information, education and communication programme interventions increases the likelihood of success. Different population groups have their own perspectives, ideas and opinions in many areas, particularly about sexual and reproductive health. Communicating effectively with them requires their direct participation;

(e) *Training of personnel.* Health professionals should be trained to cater to the special needs of the populations they serve, in such areas as interpersonal communication, sexuality, counselling and team-building, in ways that will promote work with social welfare workers, teachers, parents and community leaders. The training of educators and student peers in educational and counselling activities should focus on techniques dealing with problem-solving, listening, non-judgmental communication, conflict resolution, decision-making, counselling and basic education, as well as on sexual and reproductive health needs.

NOTES

[1]The surveys conducted under the Demographic and Health Surveys programme use a broad definition of marriage because the primary purpose of collecting the data is to provide an indicator of the beginning of exposure to reproduction. Marriage is defined as including all stable sexual relationships, regardless of the legal status of the union. Thus, women in both formal and informal unions are considered "in union" or married. Despite this broad definition of marriage, cultural differences in the way unions are formed, their social significance and their relation to child-bearing may affect the way union status and the timing of first unions are reported (IRD/Macro System, 1990).

[2]Unsafe abortion is defined as a procedure for terminating an unwanted pregnancy either by persons lacking the necessary skills or in an environment lacking the minimal medical standards or both (based on WHO, 1992).

[3]General Assembly resolution 2200A (XXI).

[4]General Assembly resolution 34/180.

REFERENCES

Alan Guttmacher Institute (1995). *Hope and Realities.* New York.

Carr, Dara, and Ann Way (1995). *Women's Lives and Experiences.* Calverton, Maryland: Macro International.

45

Council of Europe (1994). *Recent Demographic Developments in Europe*. Strasbourg, France.

European Commission (1994). *The Demographic Situation in the European Union: 1994 Report*. Strasbourg, France.

Institute for Resource Development/Macro System (1990). *An Assessment of DHS-1 Data Quality*. Demographic and Health Surveys Methodological Reports, No. 1. Columbia, Maryland.

Japan, Ministry of Health and Welfare (1995). *Latest Demographic Statistics*. Tokyo.

Larsen, Ulla (1994). Sterility in sub-Saharan Africa. *Population Studies* (London), vol. 48, No. 3 (November), pp. 459-474.

Robey, Bryant, and others (1992). *The Reproductive Revolution: New Survey Findings*. Population Reports, Series M, No. 11. Baltimore, Maryland: The Johns Hopkins University, School of Hygiene and Public Health, Population Information Program.

United Nations (1992). *Abortion Policies: A Global Review*, vol. I, *Afghanistan to France*. Sales No. E.92.XIII.8.

_____ (1993). *Abortion Policies: A Global Review*, vol. II, *Gabon to Norway*. Sales No. E.94.XIII.2.

_____ (1995a). *Report of the International Conference on Population and Development, Cairo, 5-13 September 1994*. Sales No. E.95.XIII.18.

_____ (1995b). *World Population Prospects: The 1994 Revision*. Sales No. E.95.XIII.16.

_____ (1995c). *Women's Education and Fertility Behaviour: Recent Evidence from the Demographic and Health Surveys*. Sales No. E.95.XIII.23.

_____ (1995d). *Abortion Policies: A Global Review*, vol. III, *Oman to Zimbabwe*. Sales No. E.95.XIII.24.

_____ (1995e). *Report of the Fourth World Conference on Women, Beijing, 4-15 September 1995*. A/CONF.177/20 and Add.1.

_____ (forthcoming). *World Population Monitoring, 1996*.

World Health Organization (1991). A tabulation of available data on prevalence of primary and secondary infertility. Programme on Maternal and Child Health and Family Planning, Division of Family Health. Geneva. WHO/MCH/91.9.

_____ (1992). The prevention and management of unsafe abortion: report of a technical working group. Geneva. WHO/MSM/92.5.

_____ (1994). The HIV/AIDS pandemic: 1994 overview. Geneva. WHO/GPA/TCO/SEF/94.4.

_____ (1995a). The current global situation of the HIV/AIDS pandemic. Geneva.

_____ (1995b). *An Overview of Selected Curable Sexually Transmitted Diseases*. Geneva.

_____ (1996). New estimates of maternal mortality. *Weekly Epidemiological Record* (Geneva), vol. 71, No. 13, pp. 97-100.

_____ (1994). *Abortion: A Tabulation of Available Data on the Frequency and Mortality of Unsafe Abortion*. 2nd ed. Geneva.

كيفية الحصول على منشورات الأمم المتحدة

يمكن الحصول على منشورات الأمم المتحدة من المكتبات ودور التوزيع في جميع أنحاء العالم . استعلم عنها من المكتبة
التي تتعامل معها أو اكتب إلى : الأمم المتحدة . قسم البيع في نيويورك أو في جنيف .

如何购取联合国出版物

联合国出版物在全世界各地的书店和经售处均有发售。请向书店询问或写信到纽约或日内瓦的
联合国销售组。

HOW TO OBTAIN UNITED NATIONS PUBLICATIONS

United Nations publications may be obtained from bookstores and distributors throughout the
world. Consult your bookstore or write to: United Nations, Sales Section, New York or Geneva.

COMMENT SE PROCURER LES PUBLICATIONS DES NATIONS UNIES

Les publications des Nations Unies sont en vente dans les librairies et les agences dépositaires
du monde entier. Informez-vous auprès de votre libraire ou adressez-vous à : Nations Unies,
Section des ventes, New York ou Genève.

КАК ПОЛУЧИТЬ ИЗДАНИЯ ОРГАНИЗАЦИИ ОБЪЕДИНЕННЫХ НАЦИЙ

Издания Организации Объединенных Наций можно купить в книжных магазинах
и агентствах во всех районах мира. Наводите справки об изданиях в вашем книжном
магазине или пишите по адресу: Организация Объединенных Наций, Секция по
продаже изданий, Нью-Йорк или Женева.

COMO CONSEGUIR PUBLICACIONES DE LAS NACIONES UNIDAS

Las publicaciones de las Naciones Unidas están en venta en librerías y casas distribuidoras en
todas partes del mundo. Consulte a su librero o diríjase a: Naciones Unidas, Sección de Ventas,
Nueva York o Ginebra.

Litho in United Nations, New York
93265—August 1996—4,820
ISBN 92-1-151307-3

United Nations publication
Sales No. E.96.XIII.11
ST/ESA/SER.A/157